ASTHMA

THINGS YOU SHOULD KNOW
(QUESTIONS AND ANSWERS)

By Rumi Michael Leigh

Introduction

I would like to thank and congratulate you for purchasing this book, " *Asthma, things you should know (questions and answers)*" series.

This book will help you understand, revise and have a good general knowledge and keywords of asthma and how it affects the lives of asthma sufferers.

Thanks again for purchasing this book, I hope you enjoy it !

Chapter 1

1) What is asthma?

- Asthma is a chronic lung disease that narrows and causes inflammation of the airways and the production of excess mucus that makes breathing difficult.

2) Could a person have an asthma attack without being asthmatic?

- Yes.

3) Is there a cure for asthma?

- No.

4) Since there is no cure for asthma, what is the goal of treatment?

- The goal of treatment is to manage and control the disease and to improve the quality of life of the asthma sufferer.

5) What are some of the triggers of asthma?

- Pet dander, smoke, dust mites, mold, perfumes, pests, dry and cold air, exercise-induced, respiratory infection, betablockers, aspirin, preservatives (sulfites), pollen, etc.

6) What are the signs and symptoms of asthma?

- Wheezing, coughing, shortness of breath, chest tightness, pain, etc.

7) What are the causes of asthma?

- Asthma is mainly caused by genetic and environmental factors.

8) Does asthma affect people of all ages?

- Yes.

9) What are the risk factors of asthma?

- Having other allergic conditions.
- Smoking or secondhand smoke.
- Overweight or obesity.
- Exposure to chemicals.
- Pollution.

10) What are some preventions of asthma attack?

- Identify and avoid asthma triggers.
- Use the peak flow meter.
- Follow attentively the doctor's treatment, prescription, medication.
- Learn the early signs of asthma attack.

Chapter 2

1) What are the types of asthma?

- Allergic and non-allergic asthma.

2) What is an allergic asthma?

- This is the type of asthma that is triggered by being exposed to allergens: pollen, pet dander, etc.

3) Who is an allergist?

- An allergist is a doctor that specializes in the diagnosis and treatment of allergies.

4) What is a non-allergic asthma?

- This is the type of asthma that could be exercise induced, caused by stress, illness, etc.

5) Is asthma a chronic illness?

- Yes.

6) What is a chronic illness?

- A chronic illness is an illness that is long-term.

7) Give examples of chronic illnesses.

-   Asthma, lupus, depression, etc.

8) Can asthma attack be fatal?

-   Yes.

9) Is food allergy a fatal risk factor for a person suffering from asthma?

-   Yes.

10) Compare the bronchi of an asthmatic person to the bronchi of a "normal" person.

-   The bronchi of an asthmatic person are always more or less inflamed.

Chapter 3

1) Can asthma symptoms disappear on their own?

- Yes, mild asthma symptoms can sometimes disappear on their own.

2) How is asthma prevented?

- Asthma cannot be prevented but its symptoms can be controlled.

3) When does asthma usually begin?

- Asthma usually begins during infancy.

4) Can you have asthma when you are at rest?

- Yes, you can have asthma even during rest.

5) Could stress induce an asthma attack?

- Yes, stress can induce an asthma attack.

6) Should people that suffer from asthma always have their treatment with them?

- Yes, even though their asthma is well controlled.

7) Can asthma patients live normal lives?

-    Yes, if their asthma is well controlled and they avoid asthma triggers.

8) Which airways are narrowed in asthma?

-    The bronchi and the bronchioles.

9) What kind of muscles surrounds the bronchi and bronchioles?

-    Smooth muscles.

10) What are the functions of the smooth muscles that surrounds the bronchi and bronchioles?

-    Dilation and constriction.

Chapter 4

1) Can laughing lead to an asthma attack?

- Yes, laughing too hard can lead to an asthma attack.

2) Is a doctor's prescription necessary for a meter-dosed inhaler?

- Yes.

3) What are comorbidities?

- This is when there is several illness or condition at the same time in addition to a main disease.

4) What are the comorbidities of asthma?

- Cancer, migraine, insomnia, depression, etc.

5) How is asthma treatment started in overweight or obese patients?

- First by a decrease in weight.

6) Could a person have an asthma attack without having an infection?

- Yes.

7) How does it help to drink a lot of water for asthma sufferers?

- Drinking lots of water helps to fluidify the mucus.

8) Should asthma sufferers stop exercising?

- No, they should warm-up for some minutes before exercising.

9) Can eczema trigger asthma?

- Yes.

10) What should asthma sufferers do if they are exercising outside on windy or cold days?

- They should wear a scarf or cover their mouth and nose with a mask and breathe through their nose in order to warm the air before it gets to the smooth muscles surrounding the bronchi and bronchioles because cold air constricts smooth muscles.

Chapter 5

1) What is a peak flow meter?

- It is a device used to control asthma.

2) What are bronchodilators?

- Bronchodilators dilate the airways. They are used as an urgent treatment during an asthma attack.

3) What are the types of bronchodilators?

- Short-acting and long-acting bronchodilator.

4) Give an example of a short-acting bronchodilator.

- Albuterol.

5) Give an example of a long-acting bronchodilator.

- Salmeterol.

6) What is Ventolin?

- It is a bronchodilator used for the treatment of asthma.

7) How long is the effect of Ventolin?

- About 5 minutes.

8) How long does the effect of Ventolin last?

- About 4 hours.

9) What is another name for albuterol?

- Ventolin.

10) What is the drug category of albuterol?

- It is a bronchodilator.

Chapter 6

1) Is albuterol a long-acting treatment?

- No, it is a short-acting treatment.

2) How long should you wait before administering two albuterol if it is needed?

- You should wait about one minute.

3) How often is it recommended to use albuterol?

- About 2 times a week.

4) What are short-acting beta agonists?

- Short-acting beta agonists are used during an asthma attack for fast relief.

5) Give an example of a short-acting beta agonist.

- Albuterol.

6) Are there side effects of albuterol?

- Yes.

7) What are some side effects of albuterol?

- Headache, nervousness, nausea, vomiting, irritation in the throat, irregular heartbeat, musculoskeletal pain, etc.

8) Can bronchodilator reversibility be absent during an asthma attack?

- Yes.

9) Are there side effects of beta agonists?

- Yes.

10) What are the possible side effects of beta agonists?

- Jitters, dysrhythmia, tachycardia, etc.

Chapter 7

1) What are long-acting beta agonists?

- They are used to control asthma for a long period of time.

2) What is an Axotide?

- It is an anti-inflammatory against asthma.

3) What is a fluticasone?

- It is a treatment used to decrease swelling of the airways.

4) What category of drugs is fluticasone?

- Fluticasone is a corticosteroid.

5) What is another name for fluticasone?

- Flovent.

6) Give an example of a fluticasone.

- Axotide.

7) What are the functions of corticosteroids?

- Corticosteroids decrease inflammation.

8) What should a person do after using fluticasone?

- The person should rinse their mouth with water and spit it out because fluticasone can irritate the mucus membranes.

9) How long should fluticasone be used?

- Fluticasone should be used for long-term asthma treatment.

10) Should fluticasone be used for emergency treatment?

- No.

Chapter 8

1) In the case of an asthma attack and you have a bronchodilator and a corticosteroid, which one do you use first and why?

- You use the bronchodilator first and then the corticosteroid because the bronchodilator permits the airways to be opened. And if the airways are not opened, the corticosteroid cannot get in to do its job to further decrease inflammation.

2) Should you use the inhaler before or after exercise?

- It depends. It varies on the individual, but be sure to always have your inhaler with you.

3) Which lymphocyte is over-stimulated in asthma?

- The T4 lymphocyte.

4) Name a commonly used medication that can trigger asthma.

- Aspirin.

5) What is the difference between COPD and an asthma attack?

- COPD is not reversible with treatment, but an asthma attack is reversible with treatment.

6) What is bronchial thermoplasty?

- This is a treatment for asthma that consists of heating of the airways and lungs with an electrode.

7) What is the effect of heat to the smooth muscles?

- Heat dilates smooth muscles.

8) What is the effect of cold to the smooth muscles?

- Cold constricts smooth muscles.

9) What is tachycardia?

- This is an increase in heart rate.

10) What is osteoporosis?

- This is an excessive loss of bone density.

Chapter 9

1) Do corticosteroids have side effects?

- Yes, when they are used regularly in long-term.

2) What are the possible side effects of long-term use of corticosteroids (especially for women)?

- Corticosteroids can cause osteoporosis for women.

3) When does osteoporosis usually occur in women?

- Osteoporosis usually occurs in women after menopause.

4) Does osteoporosis affect men?

- Yes, a small percentage but it is more frequent with women.

5) What is the benefit of appropriate treatment of asthma for pregnant women?

- To prevent low weight of the born baby.
- To prevent the baby from being deprived of oxygen when the mother has an asthma attack.

6) What is preeclampsia?

\-   It is a pregnancy complication that includes high blood pressure and protein in the urine.

7) What is the best treatment for preeclampsia?

\-   The best treatment is to deliver the baby.

8) What do we usually do with an inhaler before we use it?

\-   We prime the inhaler.

9) How is an inhaler primed?

\-   It is primed by shaking it and then we make some empty sprays.

10) Name the principal reasons why we prime the inhaler before use.

\-   If it is the first-time use.
\-   If it is dropped.
\-   Seven days or more without use.
\-   When it is cleaned.

Chapter 10

1) What should you check before using an inhaler?

- The same like all medications, you should check the expiry date and the number of doses.

2) What are nebulizers?

- It is a device that turns medicine into a mist that is then inhaled into the lungs. It is used for asthma treatment and other respiratory diseases.

3) Is a doctor's prescription necessary for a nebulizer?

- Yes.

4) In what situation is a nebulizer usually prescribed?

- A nebulizer is usually prescribed to people (infants, children, the elderly) who have difficulty coordinating the right usage of an inhaler for asthma treatment.

5) What kind of medicines are used in nebulizers?

- Albuterol, budesonide, etc.

6) What are the advantages of a metered-dose inhaler?

- It takes little time to administer (some seconds to a minute).
- It is portable. You can carry it with you, in your pocket, bag, etc.
- It is easy to maintain and clean.
- It is cheap.
- You don't need (power), electricity or batteries to make it function.
- It is not noisy.

7) What are the disadvantages of a metered-dose inhaler?

- It may be difficult to use correctly for infants, children, etc.

8) What are the advantages of a nebulizer?

- It is easy to use (the patient or person just have to breathe normally).

9) What are the disadvantages of a nebulizer inhaler?

- It takes a long time (over 10 minutes).
- It is not very convenient to carry with you.
- More effort is necessary to clean and maintain.
- It is expensive.
- You need electricity or battery to make it function.
- It is noisy.

10) Which has lesser side effects; a metered-dose inhaler or a nebulizer?

-   A metered-dose inhaler.

Conclusion

Thank you again for purchasing this book. I hope it has helped you in your journey to understanding asthma and how it affects the people around you who suffer from it.

Thank you.